Sepsis Awareness: A Comprehensive Guide for CNAs, PCAs, and MA's

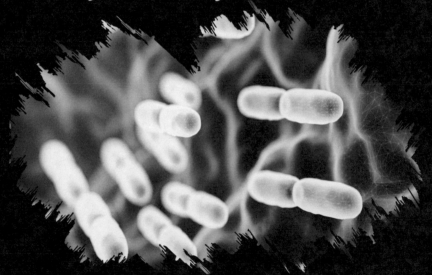

Andrea Grace Avis Patterson, BSN, RN

Table of Contents

Andrea G. A Patterson

COPYRIGHT PAGE

TITLE: SEPSIS AWARNESS: A COMPREHENSIVE GUIDE FOR CNAS, PCAS, AND MA'S

AUTHOR: ANDREA GRACE AVIS PATTERSON

Andrea G. A Patterson

DISCLAIMER:

CONTACT INFORMATION:

ANDREA@BLAZEBEAUTYBOUTIQUEB3.COM

FIRST EDITION: 2024

Procalcitonin Test

Andrea G. A Patterson

DEDICATION

This book is dedicated to my mother, Grace Mae Moore Patterson. She is the driving force behind this content. I entrusted her care to a nursing home, and they failed her. She was admitted to a facility for rehabilitation, and tragically, she passed away from an infected decubitus ulcer. Her loss deepened my passion for teaching. I am committed to educating others to help prevent the heartache of losing a loved one to an untimely death. I also aim to raise awareness about early detection and treatment, so no one else has to endure the fatal consequences of neglect.

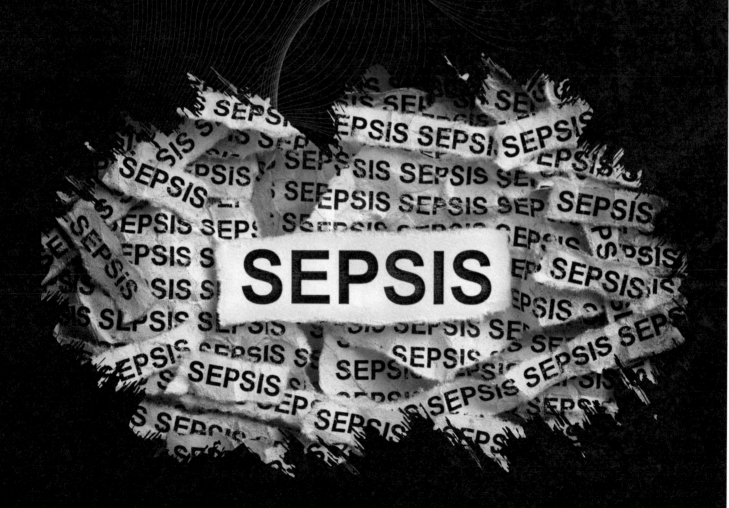

HEY, I'M ANDREA

I have worked in healthcare for over 30 years, climbing the ladder of success and cherishing every step along the way. Each role has shaped me into the loving, caring, and compassionate nurse you see today. I started as a CNA, then advanced to an LPN, and later became an RN. Currently, I work as a clinical instructor and a cardiac telemetry nurse while pursuing my MSN as a Nurse Educator. This journey has been both challenging and rewarding, and it continues to fuel my passion for teaching and patient care.

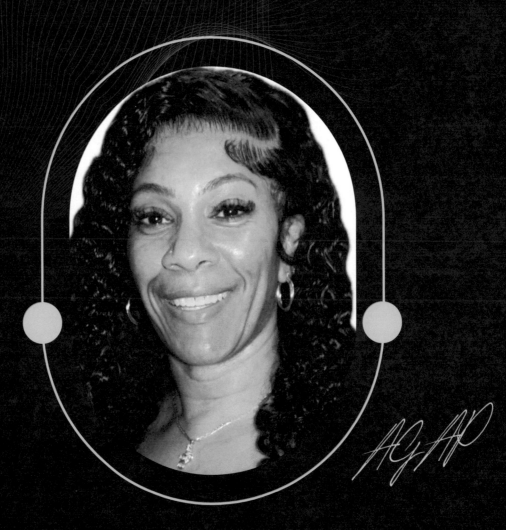

Andrea G. A Patterson

Welcome To the Course

In this book, I aim to share my knowledge as a nurse with over 25 years of experience, As a proud African American and Native American nurse, I am passionate about empowering CNAs with the skills and knowledge needed to recognize and report critical symptoms, including those associated with sepsis. My goal is to equip you with essential tools to improve patient care and outcomes, in all facilities, especially in nursing home settings.

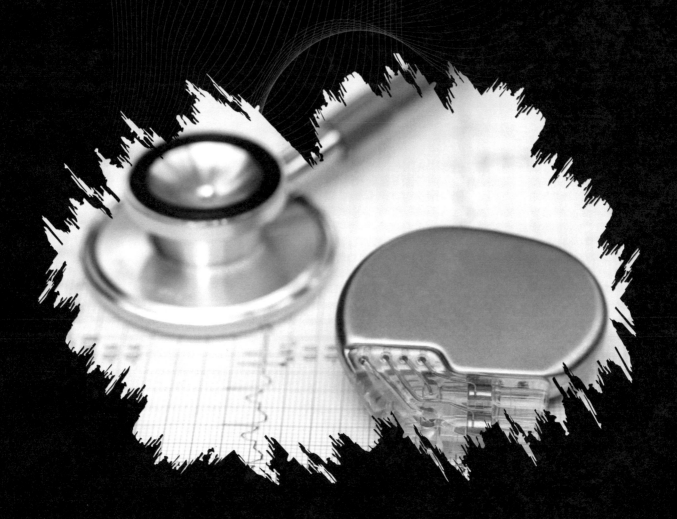

Andrea G. A Patterson

Chapter 1: Introduction to Sepsis

Definition and Overview

Sepsis is a life-threatening condition that every healthcare professional must be vigilant about. It occurs when the body's immune response to an infection becomes dysregulated, leading to widespread inflammation. If left untreated, this can result in tissue damage, organ failure, and, ultimately, death. Early detection and prompt treatment are critical to improving outcomes.

In simpler terms, sepsis is the body's response to an infection gone awry. Instead of protecting the body, the immune system overreacts, damaging healthy tissues and organs. Early intervention is vital—what may begin as a manageable infection can escalate into life-threatening sepsis within hours. In nursing homes, where the elderly are particularly vulnerable, recognizing the signs of sepsis early can make the difference between a full recovery and a tragic outcome.

Certified Nursing Assistants (CNAs) often serve as the first line of defense. Because they are frequently the first to notice changes in a resident's condition, their role in early detection cannot be overstated. Their vigilance in spotting subtle signs can help prevent sepsis from progressing to a critical stage.

Andrea G. A Patterson

Statistics and Impact on the Elderly Population

Sepsis is one of the leading causes of death in hospitals, and its impact on the elderly is especially profound. In the United States, over 1.7 million people are affected by sepsis each year, with at least 350,000 dying as a result (CDC, 2024). For the elderly, who often have compromised immune systems and multiple chronic conditions, the risk of developing sepsis is even higher.

In nursing homes, where many residents are already dealing with ongoing infections and multiple health concerns, the situation becomes even more concerning. These statistics underscore the importance of early recognition and intervention. CNAs are crucial in this process, as their ability to identify and report the early signs of sepsis can save lives.

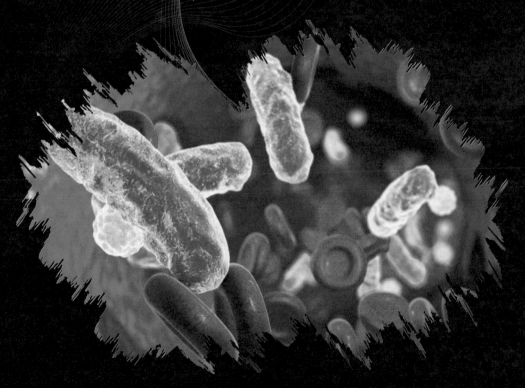

Andrea G. A Patterson

Key Takeaways:

- Sepsis occurs when the body's immune system overreacts to an infection, causing widespread inflammation that can lead to organ failure and death.

- Early detection and treatment of sepsis are crucial to improving patient outcomes.

- In nursing homes, CNAs play a vital role in recognizing the early signs of sepsis.

- The elderly are at a higher risk for sepsis due to weakened immune systems and chronic conditions.

- Statistics highlight the severity of sepsis, with over 1.7 million cases in the U.S. each year and a high mortality rate, especially among the elderly.

Reflection Question:

You are caring for an elderly patient who shows signs of confusion, increased heart rate, and mild fever. What are the first steps you would take to ensure the patient receives proper care?

Andrea G. A Patterson

What is Sepsis?

Sepsis is a severe and life-threatening condition that occurs when an infection causes the body's immune system to go into overdrive, triggering a widespread inflammatory response. This immune reaction can lead to tissue damage, organ failure, and, if left untreated, death. Essentially, the body's defense system begins to attack not only the infection but also its own tissues and organs.

Causes and Risk Factors

· Sepsis can stem from various infections, with common sources including bacterial infections, pneumonia, urinary tract infections (UTIs), and infected wounds. Any infection that is not controlled has the potential to escalate into sepsis. Certain groups are more at risk than others:

· Age: Elderly individuals are particularly vulnerable due to weakened immune systems.

· Chronic Illnesses: Conditions like diabetes, kidney disease, and lung disease increase the risk.

· Immunocompromised Individuals: Those with compromised immune systems are at higher risk.

· Invasive Devices: Devices such as catheters or IV lines can introduce infections directly into the body, heightening the risk of sepsis.

Andrea G. A Patterson

Stages of Sepsis Progression

Understanding how sepsis progresses is vital for early intervention. Sepsis typically progresses through the following stages:

1. Sepsis:

The initial stage where an infection causes a systemic inflammatory response. Symptoms may include fever, rapid heart rate, and increased breathing rate. This stage is often marked by subtle changes in the patient's condition, making early recognition crucial.

2. Severe Sepsis:

If sepsis is not treated promptly, it can progress to severe sepsis, where organ dysfunction begins. At this stage, vital organs such as the kidneys, liver, or lungs may start to fail. This is a critical phase that requires immediate medical attention to prevent further deterioration.

3. Septic Shock:

The most severe stage of sepsis, septic shock occurs when the body's blood pressure drops to dangerously low levels, even with fluid resuscitation. This stage is life-threatening and requires urgent medical intervention to stabilize the patient.

Andrea G. A Patterson

Key Takeaways:

- Sepsis is the body's overreaction to an infection, leading to widespread inflammation that can cause organ failure and death.

- Early detection and intervention are crucial to preventing the progression of sepsis.

- The most common causes of sepsis are bacterial infections, including pneumonia, urinary tract infections, and infected wounds.

- Risk factors for sepsis include age (especially the elderly), weakened immune systems, chronic illnesses, and invasive medical devices.

- Sepsis progresses through three stages: sepsis, severe sepsis, and septic shock, with septic shock being life-threatening and requiring immediate medical attention.

Reflection Question:

A patient shows symptoms of fever, rapid heart rate, and increased breathing. You are concerned it may be early sepsis. What are the immediate steps you should take to assess the situation and communicate with the medical team?

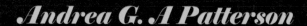
Andrea G. A Patterson

Chapter 3:
Recognizing the Signs and Symptoms of Sepsis

Early Signs of Sepsis

When it comes to spotting sepsis early, we need to be constantly vigilant. Early signs can be subtle, yet they are critical to identify and act upon. Key indicators include a sudden fever or, conversely, an abnormally low body temperature. Residents might also show a rapid heart rate or begin breathing faster than usual. Sometimes, they may appear confused or disoriented unexpectedly. These early symptoms represent the body's first warning signals, and recognizing them early can make a life-saving difference.

Progression to Severe Sepsis

If sepsis isn't identified in its early stages, it can progress quickly, and the symptoms become more severe. Watch for severe shortness of breath, extreme pain or discomfort, and a drop in urine output, which may indicate kidney issues. Changes in the skin, such as becoming clammy, sweaty, or even mottled in appearance, are also key indicators. At this stage, the situation is critical, and immediate medical intervention is essential to prevent further deterioration.

Andrea G. A Patterson

Flowchart:
Recognizing and Responding to Sepsis

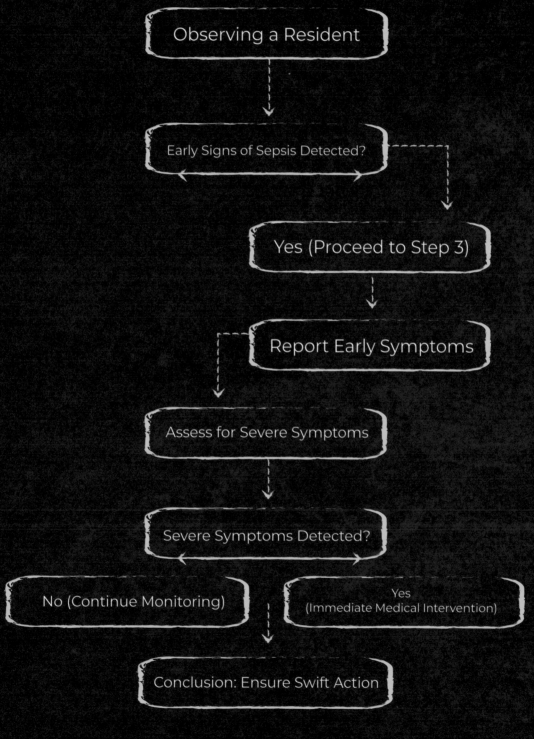

Observing a Resident

Early Signs of Sepsis Detected?

Yes (Proceed to Step 3)

Report Early Symptoms

Assess for Severe Symptoms

Severe Symptoms Detected?

No (Continue Monitoring)

Yes
(Immediate Medical Intervention)

Conclusion: Ensure Swift Action

Andrea G. A Patterson

Recognizing Sepsis in Elderly Residents

Sepsis may manifest differently in older adults, making it essential to understand these nuances. Elderly residents may not develop a high fever, even when fighting a serious infection. Instead, they often show signs of confusion or delirium more prominently—symptoms that can sometimes be mistaken for other age-related cognitive issues. Pay close attention to any sudden changes in mental status or an overall decline in condition, as these may signal an underlying infection.

Our elderly residents are especially susceptible to sepsis due to weakened immune systems and chronic health conditions, making constant vigilance a necessity. By being aware of these signs and symptoms, we can act swiftly, ensuring that our residents receive the care they need before it's too late.

Andrea G. A Patterson

Key Takeaways:

·Early signs of sepsis include fever (or low body temperature), rapid heart rate, fast breathing, and confusion.

· As sepsis progresses, more severe symptoms such as difficulty breathing, decreased urine output, and skin changes (e.g., mottling) can occur.

· Sepsis in the elderly may present with confusion or delirium rather than the typical fever response.

· CNAs play a vital role in identifying early symptoms and reporting them promptly to medical staff.

Scenario Analysis:

You are caring for an elderly patient who suddenly becomes confused, has a rapid heart rate, and shows signs of rapid breathing. What would be your immediate course of action to assess and report these symptoms?

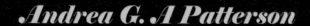

Andrea G. A Patterson

Chapter 4:
Assessing and Monitoring

Understanding the importance of vital signs is crucial in spotting sepsis early. Temperature is a primary indicator: a high fever or, conversely, an unusually low body temperature can be an initial red flag. Next is the heart rate—a rapid heart rate is often a sign that something is amiss. Respiratory rate is also essential; fast breathing can indicate that the body is struggling. Blood pressure is critical too; low blood pressure can be a sign of septic shock. Finally, oxygen saturation levels reveal how effectively the body is receiving oxygen. These vital signs provide essential clues about the body's condition and help us respond swiftly to potential sepsis.

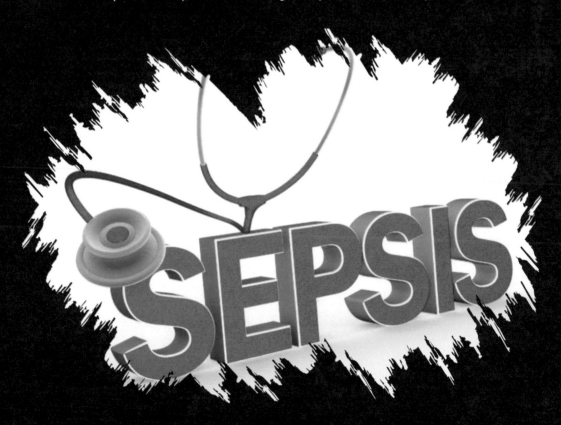

Andrea G. A Patterson

Stage	Symptoms	CNA's Role
Sepsis	Fever, rapid heart rate, chills	Monitor closely, report
Severe Sepsis	Organ dysfunction, confusion	Immediate medical alert
Septic Shock	Low blood pressure, unconsciousness	Emergency response

Andrea G. A Patterson

Utilizing MEWS for Systematic Assessment

Tools like the Modified Early Warning Score (MEWS) enable us to systematically assess a patient's condition by scoring their vital signs. It's like a quick-reference tool that helps us spot early signs of deterioration. A higher MEWS score indicates a greater need for close observation and potential escalation of care. This simple scoring method guides us in deciding when to involve medical assistance, enabling a timely response that can be critical in preventing sepsis progression.

The Role of Regular Monitoring and Documentation

Consistent monitoring and documentation are our frontline defenses against sepsis. Keeping a close watch on vital signs and documenting any changes helps us catch early warning signs. Regular monitoring allows us to track trends and notice issues before they escalate into crises. Accurate documentation is also key for communicating with the healthcare team, ensuring everyone is informed about a patient's condition. By staying vigilant and proactive, we can safeguard our residents, catching sepsis early and securing the necessary care.

Andrea G. A Patterson

Key Takeaways:

· Monitoring temperature, heart rate, respiratory rate, blood pressure, and oxygen saturation are critical in identifying early sepsis.

·Using the Modified Early Warning Score (MEWS) helps systematically assess patient risk and signals when to escalate care.

· Regular monitoring and accurate documentation of changes allow the healthcare team to act swiftly, improving patient outcomes.

Scenario Question:

Mrs. Ellis has a fever (101.5°F), elevated heart rate (105 bpm), low blood pressure (90/60 mmHg), and low oxygen saturation (90%). What are your concerns, and what actions would you take?

Chapter 5:
Effective Communication

When communicating urgent concerns, it's crucial to stay calm but assertive. This ensures the urgency is understood without creating unnecessary alarm. Clear and effective communication with the nursing team is essential. Be confident and precise when sharing observations—remember, as the eyes and ears on the front lines, your input is invaluable.

Using SBAR for Structured Communication

The SBAR method (Situation, Background, Assessment, and Recommendation) provides a clear structure for communicating effectively:

1. Situation:
Describe the immediate concern or change.

2. Background:
Provide relevant history or context.

3. Assessment:
Share your observations and any vital sign changes.

4. Recommendation:
Suggest actions or escalate as needed.

Andrea G. A Patterson

Flowchart:
Effective Communication Using SBAR and Reporting Guidelines

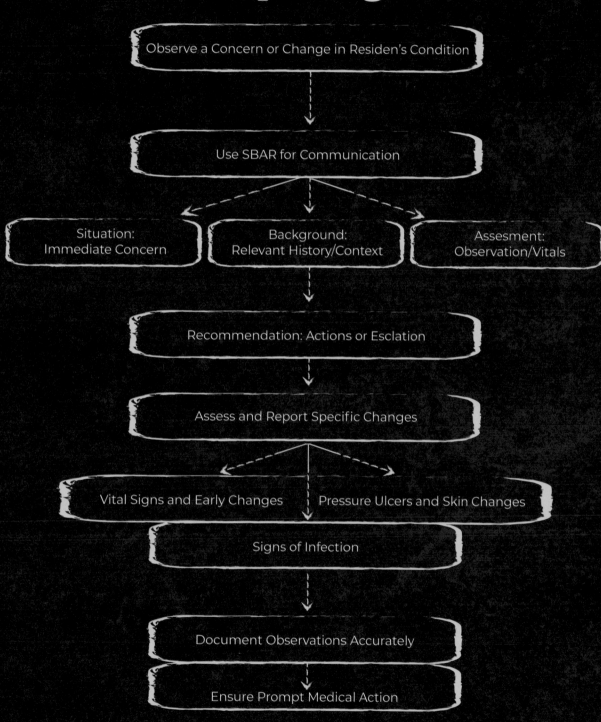

Observe a Concern or Change in Residen's Condition

Use SBAR for Communication

Situation:
Immediate Concern

Background:
Relevant History/Context

Assesment:
Observation/Vitals

Recommendation: Actions or Esclation

Assess and Report Specific Changes

Vital Signs and Early Changes | Pressure Ulcers and Skin Changes

Signs of Infection

Document Observations Accurately

Ensure Prompt Medical Action

Andrea G. A Patterson

When and What to Report

1. Vital Signs and EarlyChanges

o Vital Signs:
Report significant changes like sudden blood pressure drops or spikes in heart rate immediately.

o Confusion or Disorientation:
Any sudden mental status change should be communicated.

o Critical Symptoms:
Severe pain, shortness of breath, clammy or mottled skin are red flags that need prompt attention.

2. Red Flags for Pressure Ulcers and Skin Changes

o Early Signs:

• Redness:
Any area with developing redness.

• Warmth:
Warm spots, particularly over bony areas, compared to surrounding skin.

• Swelling and Pain:
Puffiness, swelling, or any pain the resident mentions, especially near pressure points.

Andrea G. A Patterson

SBAR Component	Purpose	Example
Situation	Clearly state the immediate concern or reason for communication.	The patient has a sudden drop in blood pressure and a high heart rate.
Background	Provide relevant context or history about the patient or situation.	The patient is 82 years old with a history of hypertension and diabetes.
Assessment	Share your observations, including any changes in vital signs or symptoms.	The patient's blood pressure is now 80/50, heart rate is 120, and they are breathing rapidly.
Recommendation	Suggest the next steps or necessary actions to address the concern.	I recommend starting fluids immediately and notifying the physician for further assessment.

Andrea G. A Patterson

When and What to Report

2. Red Flags for Pressure Ulcers and Skin Changes

• Ulcer Growth:
Any increase in ulcer size signals worsening.

• Color Changes:
Changes in skin or ulcer color.

• Drainage:
Watch for changes in fluid drainage—amount, color, or consistency.

3. Signs of Infection

o Pus or Foul Odor:
Both are indicators of infection in ulcers.

o Increased Pain and Fever:
Worsening pain or the presence of fever should be reported immediately.

o Redness Spread:
If redness starts to spread beyond the ulcer, it's a serious sign.

Accurate Documentation

Note every change with as much detail as possible, including date and time. Describe what you see, feel, and hear to provide clarity for the nursing staff.

By following these guidelines, we can ensure prompt action and prevent the escalation of potential sepsis cases. Clear communication and accurate documentation are key to keeping our residents safe and ensuring they receive timely care.

Andrea G. A Patterson

Key Takeaways:

• Urgent concerns should be communicated calmly but assertively to ensure others grasp the urgency without causing alarm.

• The SBAR (Situation, Background, Assessment, Recommendation) framework structures communication for better understanding and response.

• Early changes in vital signs, pressure ulcers, and signs of infection need immediate reporting, while precise documentation helps the healthcare team respond effectively.

Scenario Question:

You notice that a patient has a fever, increased heart rate, and rapid breathing. They also report feeling disoriented. Using the SBAR method, how would you communicate these findings to the nursing team?

Andrea G. A Patterson

Chapter 6:
Preventing Sepsis

Infection Control Practices

Preventing sepsis begins with strong infection control practices. The foundation of these practices is diligent hand hygiene. This includes thoroughly washing hands and using hand sanitizer regularly—not only for ourselves but also encouraging residents and visitors to do the same. Additionally, the proper use of personal protective equipment (PPE), such as gloves and masks, is essential in preventing the spread of infections. Ensuring that we clean and disinfect surfaces and equipment consistently is also crucial.

Infection prevention is the first line of defense against sepsis. One key area to focus on is incontinent care. Prompt attention to urinary incontinence can prevent urinary tract infections (UTIs), which, if left untreated, can lead to sepsis. This practice also helps avoid contamination of decubitus ulcers (pressure sores), which may further complicate the patient's condition.

Proper Wound Care and Hygiene

Proper wound care is another critical element in preventing infections that could lead to sepsis. For any cuts, sores, or surgical sites, it is essential to keep them clean and covered. If you notice any signs of infection—such as redness, swelling, or discharge—immediately report these changes to the nurse.

Andrea G. A Patterson

Flowchart:
Steps to Prevent Sepsis

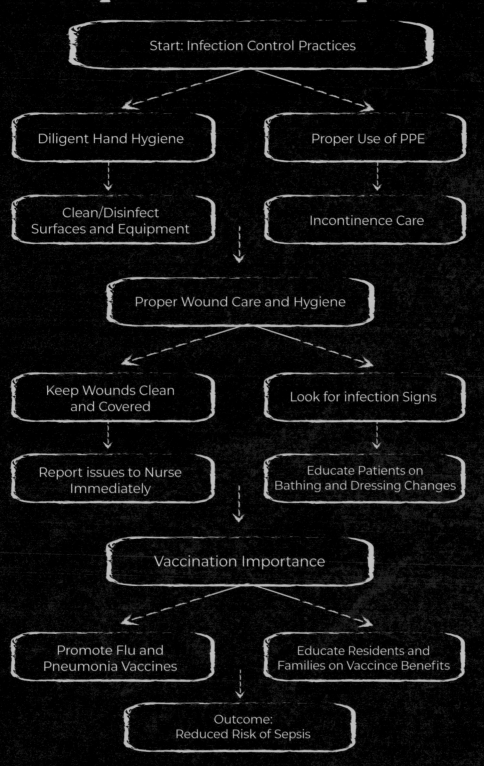

Start: Infection Control Practices

Diligent Hand Hygiene

Proper Use of PPE

Clean/Disinfect Surfaces and Equipment

Incontinence Care

Proper Wound Care and Hygiene

Keep Wounds Clean and Covered

Look for infection Signs

Report issues to Nurse Immediately

Educate Patients on Bathing and Dressing Changes

Vaccination Importance

Promote Flu and Pneumonia Vaccines

Educate Residents and Families on Vaccince Benefits

Outcome: Reduced Risk of Sepsis

Andrea G. A Patterson

Wound Care

If a dressing comes off a wound, alert the nurse so it can be re-applied promptly. While some patients may resist dressing changes, it is important to educate them about the significance of personal hygiene. Regular bathing and dressing changes are essential for preventing infections. A little extra care goes a long way in reducing the risk of complications.

Importance of Vaccination

Vaccinations are another key component in preventing sepsis, especially among elderly residents. Vaccines for flu and pneumonia are particularly important, as these infections can quickly escalate into sepsis. Encouraging and facilitating vaccinations helps protect residents from these common yet potentially deadly illnesses.

Make sure both residents and their families are well-informed about the benefits of staying up to date with vaccinations. Being proactive in this area is one of the most effective ways to safeguard their health and prevent the development of sepsis.

Andrea G. A Patterson

Key Takeaways:

· Strong infection control practices, such as hand hygiene and proper PPE use, are essential in preventing sepsis.

· Prompt incontinent care and proper hygiene can prevent urinary tract infections and other complications that may lead to sepsis.

· Proper wound care, including regular dressing changes, is crucial in preventing infection and sepsis.

· Vaccinations, particularly for flu and pneumonia, play a vital role in preventing sepsis, especially among the elderly.

Scenario Question:

You are providing care for a resident who refuses to allow their wound dressing to be changed. How would you approach the situation to ensure the dressing is changed without causing distress to the resident?

Andrea G. A Patterson

Chapter 7:
Understanding Your Role

As CNAs, PCAs, and MAs, you are the frontline caregivers—the ones who spend the most time with residents and patients. Your responsibilities are vast and essential, ranging from assisting with daily activities and ensuring comfort to monitoring health status. Beyond these tasks, you play a critical role in spotting early signs of conditions like sepsis. It's your job to be observant, attentive, and proactive in identifying changes in residents' conditions.

Nursing assistants are the eyes and ears of the healthcare team, and your contribution to early detection of sepsis is invaluable. By closely monitoring vital signs and recognizing symptoms such as fever, rapid breathing, or sudden confusion, you help catch sepsis before it escalates. Immediate reporting of these changes ensures that the healthcare team can act quickly.

Timely and accurate documentation of symptoms and any changes in residents' conditions is vital for effective management. When you act promptly, you help ensure residents receive the treatment they need in time, which can be lifesaving.

Working as part of the healthcare team means you're not alone in the fight against sepsis. Communication and collaboration with nurses, doctors, and other healthcare professionals are key. Tools like SBAR (Situation, Background, Assessment,Recommendation) enable you to communicate effectively, making sure your observations and concerns are clear and acted upon.

Andrea G. A Patterson

Being a CNA is more than just a job—it's about making a real difference in the lives of those you care for. By understanding your responsibilities, contributing to early detection and management of sepsis, and collaborating closely with the healthcare team, you ensure that residents receive the best care possible. Your role in sepsis management is essential to the health and safety of those you serve, highlighting the vital part you play in their lives.

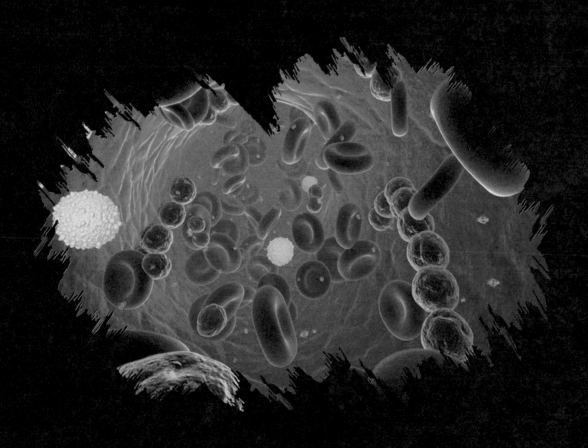

Andrea G. A Patterson

Key Takeaways:

· CNAs, PCAs, and MAs are essential in the early detection and management of sepsis.

· Early signs of sepsis, such as fever, rapid breathing, or confusion, should be reported immediately.

· Timely and accurate documentation ensures the healthcare team has the information needed to make decisions.

· Collaboration with the entire healthcare team, using tools like SBAR, ensures effective communication.

· Your proactive role can significantly improve patient outcomes, making your work an essential part of sepsis management.

Scenario Question:

You notice a resident has a fever, rapid breathing, and confusion. What immediate actions should you take to assess the situation and communicate with the healthcare team?

Andrea G. A Patterson

Chapter 8:
Scenarios - Real-Life Applications of Sepsis Detection

In this chapter, we will explore real-life examples of sepsis cases in nursing homes to understand the crucial role CNAs play in detecting and responding to sepsis. We'll use the SBAR (Situation, Background, Assessment, Recommendation) communication method to demonstrate how CNAs can effectively communicate changes in patient condition, ensuring timely intervention.

Using SBAR for Clear Communication

Situation:
Briefly describe the current situation.
Example:
"Mr. Johnson's heart rate has suddenly increased to 120 beats per minute."

Background:
Provide relevant context or background information.
Example:
"He was admitted with a urinary tract infection three days ago."

Assessment:
Share your professional assessment of the situation.
Example:
"He's also showing signs of confusion, and his skin feels clammy."

Andrea G. A Patterson

Recommendation:

State the recommended course of action.

Example: "I recommend that we check his vitals again immediately and alert the on-call physician."

Using SBAR helps us communicate clearly and concisely, ensuring that no detail is overlooked and that residents receive the timely care they need. It allows CNAs to be professional, thorough, and proactive in their role, ensuring their voice is heard within the healthcare team.

Real-life Examples of Sepsis Cases in Nursing Homes

Now, let's examine some real-life scenarios to understand how early detection and proactive reporting can save lives.

Case Study 1: Mrs. Smith

Mrs. Smith, an 85-year-old resident, had been recovering from a urinary tract infection. One afternoon, you noticed she seemed more confused than usual, wasn't as responsive, and her skin felt clammy. Her heart rate was elevated, and you immediately reported these changes to the nurse.

Action Taken:

The nurse contacted the provider, and they ordered a sepsis workup.

Thanks to your quick actions, Mrs. Smith received the necessary antibiotics and fluids, and her condition improved.

Andrea G. A Patterson

This case highlights the importance of being observant and proactive in preventing the progression of sepsis.

Case Study 2: Mr. Johnson

Mr. Johnson, a 90-year-old with diabetes, had a wound on his foot that wasn't healing well. During routine checks, you noticed the area around the wound was becoming red and swollen, and Mr. Johnson had a fever.

Action Taken:

You reported your findings immediately, and further tests confirmed that he was developing sepsis. Early intervention with antibiotics and wound care helped prevent the infection from spreading. Your attention to detail and timely reporting were key to his recovery.

Scenario 1: Sudden Confusion in Mrs. Brown

Imagine you're checking on Mrs. Brown, an 82-year-old resident. She is usually cheerful and chatty, but today she seems confused and disoriented. Her temperature is slightly elevated, and she's breathing rapidly.

Action:

· Report her symptoms to the nurse immediately.

· Monitor her vital signs closely, documenting any changes.

· Ensure that the nurse has all necessary information for further action.

Scenario 2: Unexplained Pain in Mr. Lee

Mr. Lee, a 78-year-old resident, complains of severe abdominal pain that started suddenly. His heart rate is high, and he feels cold to the touch.

Action:

·Alert the nurse immediately, as these could be signs of sepsis.

· Ensure Mr. Lee is comfortable and keep monitoring his condition.

· Document all observations clearly for the medical team's review.

Scenario 3: Wound Infection in Mr. Davis

During a routine check, you notice that Mr. Davis's surgical wound is red, swollen, and has a foul-smelling discharge. He also has a fever.

Andrea G. A Patterson

Scenario 4: Mrs. Thompson's Urinary Symptoms

Mrs. Thompson, an 82-year-old resident, has a fever of 101°F, a rapid heart rate of 110 beats per minute, and is more confused than usual. She also complains of a burning sensation while urinating.

Questions:

· What are the potential signs of sepsis in Mrs. Thompson?

· What immediate actions should you take as a CNA?

· How would you communicate your concerns to the nursing staff?

Answers:

· Potential Signs of Sepsis: Mrs. Thompson is showing several potential signs of sepsis, including a fever, a rapid heart rate, confusion, and symptoms of a urinary tract infection.

• Immediate Actions:
As a CNA, you should monitor her vital signs closely, ensure her comfort, and promptly report all symptoms to the nurse.

• Communicating Concerns:
When communicating with the nursing staff, be clear and concise. Mention the specific signs and symptoms you've observed, emphasizing the urgency due to the risk of sepsis. Provide a detailed account to help guide the next steps.

Practicing these scenarios helps us prepare for real-life situations. Our role in early detection and response is vital, and by being prepared, we can provide the best care for our patients/residents.

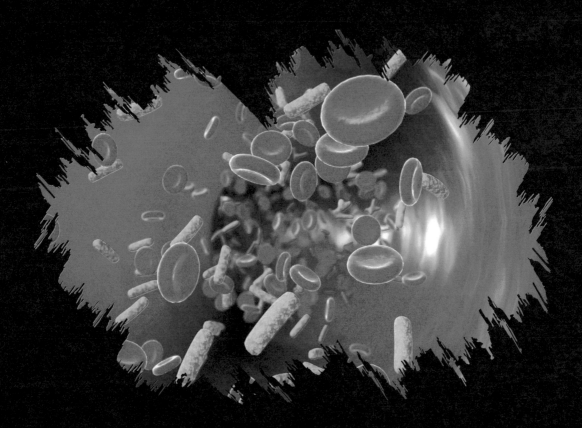

Andrea G. A Patterson

Key Takeaways:

· The SBAR method is an effective tool for clear and concise communication about a patient's condition.

· Early detection of sepsis in nursing home residents is critical for timely intervention and treatment.

· Observing changes in mental status, vital signs, and wound conditions can help identify potential cases of sepsis.

· CNAs play an essential role in detecting sepsis and ensuring residents receive prompt, life-saving care.

Reflection Question:

A resident exhibits confusion, rapid breathing, and fever. You suspect sepsis. What are your first steps? Consider how you would document and communicate this to the medical team. Practice using SBAR to organize your thoughts and ensure accurate reporting.

Andrea G. A Patterson

Websites

Explore these trusted websites for comprehensive information on sepsis:

• Centers for Disease Control and Prevention (CDC): The CDC provides up-to-date information, guidelines, and resources on sepsis prevention and management.

•Sepsis Alliance: This organization is dedicated to raising awareness about sepsis, providing educational resources, and supporting survivors and their families.

Resources and References

Reading Materials

For those looking to dive deeper into sepsis, here are some recommended reading materials:

• "Surviving Sepsis Campaign Guidelines" by the Society of Critical Care Medicine and the European Society of Intensive Care Medicine

• "Sepsis and Septic Shock: A History" by R. Phillip Dellinger and Mitchell M. Levy

•"Textbook of Sepsis" edited by Jean-Louis Vincent

Centers for Disease Control and Prevention (CDC). (2024). About Sepsis. U.S. Department of Health and Human Services. Retrieved from CDC Sepsis Overview.

Andrea G. A Patterson

Glossary

1. Sepsis:
A serious infection that causes the body to attack itself, leading to organ damage.

2. Infection:
When germs like bacteria or viruses invade the body and cause illness.

3. Septic Shock:
The most severe stage of sepsis, where blood pressure drops, and organs may stop working.

4. Vital Signs:
Basic body measurements like temperature, heart rate, and breathing rate, used to monitor health.

5. Fever:
A body temperature higher than normal, often a sign of infection.

6. Hypothermia:
An unusually low body temperature, which can sometimes indicate sepsis.

7. Tachycardia:
A fast heart rate, which could mean the body is fighting an infection.

8. Tachypnea:
Fast breathing, often seen in people with sepsis.

9. Blood Pressure:
The force of blood against the arteries. Low blood pressure in sepsis can be a warning sign.

10. Lactate:
A substance that increases when the body isn't getting enough oxygen; high levels may signal sepsis.

11. Antibiotics:
Medicines used to fight infections caused by bacteria.

Andrea G. A Patterson

12. IV (Intravenous):
A way to deliver fluids and medicines directly into the
bloodstream.
13. Organ Failure:
When organs like the heart, lungs, or kidneys stop
working due to illness.
14. Inflammation:
Swelling or redness in the body as it fights infection; too
much inflammation can harm the body in sepsis.
15. Immune System:
The body's defense system that fights infections.
16. Cytokines:
Small proteins that help the immune system but can
cause inflammation when out of control.
17. Blood Culture:
A test to find bacteria in the blood, used to diagnose
infections.
18. Shock:
A dangerous condition where blood flow drops, making
it hard for the body to function.
19. Pain and Discomfort:
Common feelings in sepsis, often in areas with infection.
20. Mental Confusion:
When someone seems confused or disoriented, which
can be a symptom of sepsis.

These terms can help CNAs understand the basics of sepsis
and recognize warning signs, improving their ability to
support patient care effectively.

Andrea G. A Patterson

Helpful Tips to Stay Organized During Your Shift

- Arrive 10-15 minutes early.
- Get your assignment and report from the previous shift.
- Start getting morning vitals and write your name on the whiteboard in each room. Report any abnormal vitals to the nurse.
- Give fresh water to patients if appropriate, and provide clean linen.
- Stock your rooms with gloves, gowns, wipes, and any other necessary supplies.
- Ensure patients are sitting up in bed during meals to prevent aspiration or spilling food.
- Know which patients need assistance with meals to ensure they receive proper support.
- Complete charting as needed.
- Team up with a co-worker to handle two-assist patients together. Once these patients are washed and up, assist one-assist and independent patients with their morning ADLs (Activities of Daily Living).
- Round on your patients every 2 hours to prevent excessive use of call bells.
- Avoid washing patients at 3 p.m. unless requested. If all your work is done in the morning, you can relax and wait for call bells to ring, if any.
- Ensure all patient needs are met early to minimize call bell use.

Andrea G. A Patterson

Inspiration

**Growing
Teamwork Makes the Dream
Work!**

Success

Andrea G. A Patterson

Your Notes

_____

_____

_____

_____

_____

_____

_____

_____

_____

_____

_____

Enjoy the process.

Andrea G. A Patterson

Made in the USA
Columbia, SC
18 February 2025

54054378R00027